The Galveston Diet

A Coastal Approach to Health and Weight Management for Vibrant Living

By

CANDICE FOSTER

TABLE OF CONTENTS

INTRODUCTION

In the realm of health and wellness, numerous diet trends come and go, each promising a path to optimal well-being. Amidst this sea of options, one stands out as a refreshing and distinctive approach – The Galveston Diet. Rooted in the coastal lifestyle of Galveston, Texas, this dietary regimen not only focuses on weight management but also emphasizes overall health and vitality.

The Galveston Diet takes inspiration from the coastal environment, integrating elements of a balanced and nourishing lifestyle that mirrors the rhythms of the sea. Developed by Dr. Mary Claire Haver, a renowned physician with a passion for empowering individuals to achieve their health goals, this diet is not just about shedding pounds but about fostering vibrant living.

The coastal influence on The Galveston Diet is palpable, as it draws on the abundance of fresh and nutrient-rich foods found in the region. Seafood, a staple in coastal communities, takes center stage in this dietary approach. Rich in omega-3 fatty acids and lean proteins, fish and shellfish become essential components for supporting heart health and cognitive function. The diet also encourages the consumption of a variety of colorful fruits and vegetables, harnessing the power of antioxidants and essential vitamins.

Beyond its focus on nutrition, The Galveston Diet recognizes the importance of mindful eating. Coastal living often involves savoring meals slowly, appreciating the flavors, and connecting with the community. This approach aims to instill a sense of mindfulness in individuals, fostering a healthier relationship with food and promoting better digestion.

One of the unique aspects of The Galveston Diet is its consideration of hormonal changes, particularly in women. Dr. Haver, drawing on her expertise in obstetrics and gynecology, has tailored the diet to address the specific needs of women as they navigate various life stages. The hormonal fluctuations that occur during perimenopause and menopause can impact metabolism and weight management, and this diet offers a nuanced approach to support women in achieving and maintaining a healthy weight.

The Galveston Diet is not a one-size-fits-all solution; instead, it encourages personalized choices based on individual preferences and health goals. It promotes the understanding that each person's body is unique, and what works for one may not work for another. By fostering this awareness, the diet empowers individuals to make informed decisions about their nutrition, leading to sustainable and long-term success in health and weight management.

In addition to its emphasis on nutrition, The Galveston Diet advocates for an active lifestyle. Coastal living often involves outdoor activities, and this dietary approach aligns with the benefits of regular exercise. Whether it's a brisk walk along the beach, cycling by the shoreline, or engaging in water sports, the diet encourages individuals to find joy in movement and incorporate physical activity into their daily routines.

The Galveston Diet also addresses the importance of community support. In coastal regions, a sense of community is integral to daily life. Similarly, this diet emphasizes the role of a supportive community in fostering a positive and sustainable approach to health.

Online forums, social media groups, and local meet-ups provide a platform for individuals following The Galveston Diet to share experiences, exchange tips, and motivate each other on their wellness journeys.

As we delve deeper into The Galveston Diet, this exploration will uncover its guiding principles, detailed dietary recommendations, and practical tips for implementation. Through a coastal lens, we will navigate the waves of nutritional choices, hormonal considerations, mindful eating practices, and the importance of an active and supportive lifestyle. Join us on this voyage towards vibrant living – where health and well-being merge seamlessly with the coastal essence of The Galveston Diet.

CHAPTER 1

Welcome to the Galveston Diet

Welcome to the Galveston Diet, a revolutionary approach to wellness that transcends conventional notions of weight loss and embraces a holistic lifestyle transformation. Galveston, a coastal gem, not only offers picturesque views but also serves as the backdrop for a nutritional philosophy that has taken the health and wellness community by storm.

At the heart of the Galveston Diet is the profound understanding that women's bodies are unique, responding differently to various dietary patterns. Dr. Mary Claire Haver, the visionary behind this paradigm shift, has crafted a comprehensive program tailored to the specific needs of women over 40. Unlike generic diets, the Galveston approach recognizes and addresses the hormonal fluctuations that often accompany this stage of life.

The cornerstone of this diet is intermittent fasting, a time-tested method that promotes metabolic flexibility and encourages the body to tap into its fat reserves for energy. Dr. Haver advocates for a 16:8 fasting window, allowing the body to enter a state of ketosis, where it burns fat efficiently. This strategic fasting is not about deprivation but rather optimizing the body's natural processes.

What sets the Galveston Diet apart is its emphasis on anti-inflammatory foods. Dr. Haver underscores the crucial role inflammation plays in weight gain and various health issues. By incorporating an array of nutrient-dense, anti-inflammatory foods, followers of the Galveston Diet nourish their bodies while fostering an environment that supports overall well-being.

The Galveston Diet isn't just about what you eat; it's a lifestyle that prioritizes self-care. Dr. Haver encourages mindful eating, emphasizing the importance of savoring each bite and listening to the body's hunger cues. This mindful approach extends beyond the plate, encouraging individuals to engage in stress-reducing activities, adequate sleep, and regular physical exercise.

Intriguingly, the Galveston Diet also delves into the science of circadian rhythms, aligning eating patterns with the body's internal clock. This synchronization not only enhances the effectiveness of the diet but also contributes to improved sleep quality and overall vitality.

The Galveston community has become a beacon of support for individuals embarking on this transformative journey. Online forums and social media groups buzz with shared experiences, success stories, and a camaraderie that reinforces the sense of community. Dr. Haver's hands-on approach, including live Q&A sessions and personalized guidance, adds a personalized touch that sets this diet apart.

Beyond the tangible benefits of weight loss, followers of the Galveston Diet report increased energy levels, mental clarity, and a renewed sense of confidence. The diet becomes a gateway to rediscovering one's relationship with food and, ultimately, with oneself.

As the Galveston Diet gains traction, it challenges prevailing notions of weight loss, offering a refreshing perspective that acknowledges the complexity of the human body. It is not a one-size-fits-all solution but a nuanced, tailored approach that resonates with the diverse needs of women navigating the intricacies of midlife.

In conclusion, the Galveston Diet transcends the realm of conventional diets, presenting a captivating fusion of science, nutrition, and lifestyle. Dr. Mary Claire Haver's innovative approach has sparked a movement that empowers women to reclaim control of their health, fostering a profound transformation that extends far beyond the numbers on a scale. Welcome to the Galveston Diet—a voyage of self-discovery, well-being, and a renewed zest for life.

Understanding the Coastal Approach

The coastal approach is an intricate tapestry of ecological, geological, and human elements, interwoven along the meeting point of land and sea. It transcends mere geographical significance, embodying a dynamic intersection where diverse forces converge, giving rise to ecosystems teeming with life, shaping geological formations, and influencing human civilizations in profound ways.

At its essence, understanding the coastal approach requires delving into the symbiotic relationship between land and sea. Coastal regions serve as ecological transition zones, where terrestrial and marine environments intertwine, creating unique habitats that support an extraordinary array of biodiversity. Mangroves, salt marshes, and tidal zones act as crucial nurseries for marine life, showcasing nature's ability to adapt and thrive in the ever-shifting balance of coastal ecosystems.

Geologically, the coastal approach provides a canvas where natural processes sculpt the earth in remarkable ways. Erosion and deposition, driven by the relentless dance of waves, carve coastlines into picturesque formations, from towering cliffs to gentle sandy shores. The constant interplay between tides, currents, and sedimentation molds landscapes over time, creating geological wonders that stand as testaments to the enduring power of nature.

Human societies have long been drawn to the coast, establishing civilizations that bear the imprint of the sea. Coastal cities, with their bustling ports and maritime traditions, epitomize the fusion of land and water in human culture. Trade routes, cultural exchanges, and economic prosperity often find their roots in these coastal hubs, illustrating the profound impact of the coastal approach on the development of human societies throughout history.

Yet, the coastal approach is not without its challenges. Rising sea levels, coastal erosion, and extreme weather events pose significant threats to both natural ecosystems and human communities. Climate change amplifies these risks, underscoring the urgency of comprehending the delicate balance inherent in coastal regions. Sustainable coastal management becomes imperative, demanding a harmonious coexistence between human activities and the preservation of these vital ecosystems.

In the pursuit of understanding the coastal approach, interdisciplinary collaboration becomes paramount. Ecologists, geologists, climatologists, and sociologists converge to unravel the complexities of this dynamic interface. Cutting-edge technologies, from satellite imagery to oceanographic research vessels, facilitate a deeper exploration of coastal dynamics, enabling scientists to monitor changes and implement effective conservation measures.

Furthermore, the coastal approach invites philosophical reflection, prompting contemplation on humanity's role as stewards of the land and sea. It challenges societies to embrace sustainable practices, fostering a holistic approach that respects the interconnectedness of ecosystems and recognizes the fragility of coastal environments.

In conclusion, the coastal approach emerges as a captivating realm where nature's forces converge with human endeavors. Understanding this intricate interplay requires a multifaceted exploration, encompassing ecological, geological, and societal dimensions. As we navigate the complex challenges posed by climate change and human activities, the coastal approach beckons us to forge a path towards harmony, preserving the richness of these dynamic landscapes for generations to come.

CHAPTER 2

The Galveston Lifestyle

The Galveston lifestyle is a unique blend of coastal charm, historical richness, and vibrant community living. Situated on the Gulf of Mexico in Texas, this island city has long been a destination for those seeking a relaxed and distinctive way of life.

One of the defining features of the Galveston lifestyle is its deep-rooted connection to maritime history. The city's port, one of the busiest in the United States, has played a pivotal role in shaping its character. The seafaring heritage is evident in the architecture, with Victorian-era buildings lining the streets, each telling a tale of the island's past. The historic district, known as The Strand, is a testament to this bygone era, offering a nostalgic journey through time with its well-preserved facades and cobblestone streets.

Beyond its historical allure, Galveston is renowned for its picturesque beaches. Miles of sandy shores stretch along the Gulf, providing residents with a year-round escape to sun and surf. The island's beaches are not only a haven for relaxation but also a hub of recreational activities. Water sports, fishing, and beachcombing are popular pastimes, creating a lifestyle deeply intertwined with the ebb and flow of the tides.

Galveston's climate contributes significantly to its appealing lifestyle. With mild winters and warm summers, residents enjoy a comfortable environment that encourages outdoor activities throughout the year. This temperate climate fosters a sense of wellbeing and facilitates a variety of community events and festivals.

The island's emphasis on community is another hallmark of the Galveston lifestyle. The close-knit neighborhoods and friendly atmosphere make it a welcoming place for newcomers and a tight bond for long-time residents. Local gatherings, farmers' markets, and cultural events enhance the sense of belonging, creating a lifestyle that values both individual tranquility and communal connection.

The culinary scene in Galveston is a delectable reflection of its coastal location. Seafood takes center stage, with fresh catches gracing the menus of local eateries. From shrimp po'boys to Gulf oysters, residents savor the flavors of the sea, creating a gastronomic experience that mirrors the island's maritime identity.

Additionally, the diverse array of dining options caters to a wide range of tastes, ensuring that everyone can find something to satisfy their palate.

Education and cultural enrichment are integral components of the Galveston lifestyle. The city boasts educational institutions that cater to diverse interests, fostering a love for learning from an early age. Museums and cultural centers showcase the island's history and art, providing residents with opportunities to engage in intellectual pursuits and artistic expression.

Despite its relatively small size, Galveston offers a wealth of recreational options. Parks and nature reserves provide spaces for outdoor enthusiasts, while a variety of sports and fitness facilities cater to those seeking an active lifestyle. The island's commitment to health and wellness is evident in the availability of walking and biking trails, promoting an ethos of physical activity and a balanced approach to life.

The Galveston lifestyle also benefits from its proximity to Houston, a major metropolitan center. This accessibility allows residents to enjoy the perks of city life while still relishing the tranquility of island living. Whether it's a weekend getaway or a cultural excursion, the connection to Houston expands the horizons of the Galveston lifestyle.

In conclusion, the Galveston lifestyle is a harmonious blend of history, nature, community, and culture. From its maritime roots to its modern amenities, the island city offers a distinctive way of life that appeals to those seeking a balance between tradition and progress, relaxation and recreation. Whether enjoying the beaches, savoring local cuisine, or embracing the community spirit, residents of Galveston find themselves immersed in a lifestyle that is both enriching and enduring.

Embracing coastal living can significantly contribute to overall health and well-being. The allure of living by the sea extends beyond picturesque landscapes and soothing waves; it encompasses a multitude of physical, mental, and emotional benefits. From the invigorating sea air to the opportunities for outdoor activities, coastal living fosters a lifestyle that promotes both physical and mental wellness.

One of the primary health advantages of coastal living is the quality of air. The sea breeze carries with it negatively charged ions, which are believed to have various positive effects on the human body. These ions are thought to increase serotonin levels, a neurotransmitter associated with mood and stress regulation. Breathing in this fresh, ion-rich air can contribute to an improved sense of well-being and mental clarity.

Moreover, coastal areas often boast cleaner air compared to urban environments. Proximity to the sea means lower pollution levels, as the ocean breeze helps disperse pollutants. This cleaner air can lead to better respiratory health, reducing the risk of respiratory issues and promoting lung function. Individuals with conditions such as asthma may find relief in the coastal environment.

In addition to the air quality, the coastal lifestyle encourages outdoor activities that support physical health. The beach serves as a natural playground for various forms of exercise, from brisk walks along the shore to more intense activities like beach volleyball or surfing. Engaging in regular physical activity has well-documented benefits for cardiovascular health, weight management, and overall fitness.

The therapeutic effects of being near the water cannot be overstated. The sound of waves crashing on the shore has a calming effect on the mind, reducing stress and promoting relaxation. This auditory experience, often referred to as "blue space," has been associated with improved mental well-being. Living by the coast provides easy access to this natural stress-reliever, allowing residents to unwind and recharge simply by taking a stroll along the beach.

Furthermore, exposure to natural light is a crucial factor in maintaining a healthy circadian rhythm and regulating sleep patterns. Coastal living offers ample sunlight, which is not only essential for the body's production of vitamin D but also contributes to better sleep quality. A well-regulated sleep cycle is linked to improved cognitive function, mood stability, and overall mental health.

The sense of community in coastal areas also plays a pivotal role in supporting well-being. Coastal living often fosters a close-knit community where residents share a common appreciation for the natural beauty surrounding them. This sense of belonging and social connection contributes to emotional health and provides a support system during challenging times.

In terms of nutrition, coastal regions often offer access to fresh and diverse seafood. Seafood is rich in omega-3 fatty acids, which are known for their numerous health benefits, including reducing the risk of heart disease, supporting brain health, and reducing inflammation. Incorporating locally sourced seafood into the diet can be a delicious and nutritious way to enhance overall health.

The mental health benefits of coastal living extend beyond the physical environment. The slower pace of life often associated with coastal communities can reduce the pressures and stressors of modern urban living. The proximity to nature provides opportunities for mindfulness and introspection, fostering a mental space conducive to relaxation and creativity.

While embracing coastal living can be a transformative experience for health, it's essential to consider potential challenges such as coastal erosion and rising sea levels. Sustainable practices and thoughtful urban planning are crucial to preserving the coastal environment and ensuring the long-term well-being of coastal communities.

In conclusion, coastal living offers a myriad of health benefits, ranging from the physical advantages of clean air and outdoor activities to the mental and emotional well-being derived from the soothing sounds of the sea and a close-knit community. Embracing coastal living is not just a lifestyle choice; it is a holistic approach to health that recognizes the interconnectedness of our well-being with the natural world around us. As individuals seek ways to enhance their overall health and quality of life, the coastal lifestyle stands out as a harmonious blend of nature, community, and well-being.

Embracing Coastal Living for Health

Embracing coastal living can significantly contribute to overall health and well-being. The allure of living by the sea extends beyond picturesque landscapes and soothing waves; it encompasses a multitude of physical, mental, and emotional benefits. From the invigorating sea air to the opportunities for outdoor activities, coastal living fosters a lifestyle that promotes both physical and mental wellness.

One of the primary health advantages of coastal living is the quality of air. The sea breeze carries with it negatively charged ions, which are believed to have various positive effects on the human body. These ions are thought to increase serotonin levels, a neurotransmitter associated with mood and stress regulation. Breathing in this fresh, ion-rich air can contribute to an improved sense of well-being and mental clarity.

Moreover, coastal areas often boast cleaner air compared to urban environments. Proximity to the sea means lower pollution levels, as the ocean breeze helps disperse pollutants. This cleaner air can lead to better respiratory health, reducing the risk of respiratory issues and promoting lung function. Individuals with conditions such as asthma may find relief in the coastal environment.

In addition to the air quality, the coastal lifestyle encourages outdoor activities that support physical health. The beach serves as a natural playground for various forms of exercise, from brisk walks along the shore to more intense activities like beach volleyball or surfing. Engaging in regular physical activity has well-documented benefits for cardiovascular health, weight management, and overall fitness.

The therapeutic effects of being near the water cannot be overstated. The sound of waves crashing on the shore has a calming effect on the mind, reducing stress and promoting relaxation. This auditory experience, often referred to as "blue space," has been associated with improved mental well-being. Living by the coast provides easy access to this natural stress-reliever, allowing residents to unwind and recharge simply by taking a stroll along the beach.

Furthermore, exposure to natural light is a crucial factor in maintaining a healthy circadian rhythm and regulating sleep patterns. Coastal living offers ample sunlight, which is not only essential for the body's production of vitamin D but also contributes to better sleep quality. A well-regulated sleep cycle is linked to improved cognitive function, mood stability, and overall mental health.

The sense of community in coastal areas also plays a pivotal role in supporting well-being. Coastal living often fosters a close-knit community where residents share a common appreciation for the natural beauty surrounding them. This sense of belonging and social connection contributes to emotional health and provides a support system during challenging times.

In terms of nutrition, coastal regions often offer access to fresh and diverse seafood. Seafood is rich in omega-3 fatty acids, which are known for their numerous health benefits, including reducing the risk of heart disease, supporting brain health, and reducing inflammation. Incorporating locally sourced seafood into the diet can be a delicious and nutritious way to enhance overall health.

The mental health benefits of coastal living extend beyond the physical environment. The slower pace of life often associated with coastal communities can reduce the pressures and stressors of modern urban living. The proximity to nature provides opportunities for mindfulness and introspection, fostering a mental space conducive to relaxation and creativity.

While embracing coastal living can be a transformative experience for health, it's essential to consider potential challenges such as coastal erosion and rising sea levels. Sustainable practices and thoughtful urban planning are crucial to preserving the coastal environment and ensuring the long-term well-being of coastal communities.

In conclusion, coastal living offers a myriad of health benefits, ranging from the physical advantages of clean air and outdoor activities to the mental and emotional well-being derived from the soothing sounds of the sea and a close-knit community. Embracing coastal living is not just a lifestyle choice; it is a holistic approach to health that recognizes the interconnectedness of our well-being with the natural world around us. As individuals seek ways to enhance their overall health and quality of life, the coastal lifestyle stands out as a harmonious blend of nature, community, and well-being.

Incorporating Local Ingredients and Flavors

In the vibrant culinary landscape of Galveston, Texas, incorporating local ingredients and flavors into the diet is not just a culinary choice but a celebration of the region's rich cultural and agricultural heritage. Nestled along the Gulf of Mexico, Galveston offers a bounty of fresh seafood, locally grown produce, and a fusion of cultural influences that have shaped its distinctive culinary identity. Embracing these local elements not only enhances the gastronomic experience but also contributes to sustainable practices and community support.

Galveston's proximity to the Gulf provides a diverse selection of fresh seafood that forms the backbone of many local dishes. From succulent Gulf shrimp to flaky red snapper, the seafood offerings are a testament to the city's connection to its maritime roots. Incorporating these treasures from the sea into the Galveston diet not only ensures a fresh and flavorful experience but also supports local fishermen and sustains the region's fishing industry.

One iconic dish that showcases Galveston's love for seafood is the classic Gulf Coast shrimp boil. Combining large Gulf shrimp, corn on the cob, and red potatoes, seasoned with a blend of local spices, this communal feast is a staple at family gatherings and community events. The aromatic blend of spices, often including Old Bay seasoning and cayenne pepper, infuses the dish with a zesty kick that reflects the bold flavors synonymous with Gulf Coast cuisine.

While seafood takes center stage, Galveston's culinary scene also draws inspiration from the diverse cultural influences that have shaped the region. The city's history includes periods of Spanish, Mexican, and Cajun influence, each leaving its mark on the local cuisine. Tex-Mex flavors, for example, are seamlessly woven into the fabric of Galveston's food culture, giving rise to dishes like seafood enchiladas and shrimp tacos that showcase a harmonious blend of Gulf ingredients with Mexican flair.

The fertile soil surrounding Galveston provides a rich tapestry of locally grown produce, further enhancing the culinary offerings. From juicy vine-ripened tomatoes to sweet Texas onions, incorporating these fresh, seasonal ingredients adds depth and vibrancy to dishes. Local farmers' markets become a treasure trove for chefs and home cooks alike, offering an array of fruits and vegetables that reflect the changing seasons.

Galveston's embrace of local flavors extends beyond the kitchen and into its beverage culture. Craft breweries and wineries in the area take advantage of the region's resources to produce unique libations that complement the local cuisine. Brews infused with Gulf-inspired ingredients, such as citrus and sea salt, or wines crafted from Texas-grown grapes, offer a taste of the terroir and a perfect pairing for seafood-centric meals.

Sustainable practices play a crucial role in Galveston's commitment to preserving its natural resources and supporting local communities. By prioritizing locally sourced ingredients, chefs and residents contribute to a more eco-friendly food system. This approach not only reduces the carbon footprint associated with transportation but also fosters a sense of community and collaboration between farmers, fishermen, and consumers.

Community-supported agriculture (CSA) programs and farm-to-table initiatives have gained popularity in Galveston, providing residents with direct access to fresh, locally grown produce. These programs not only strengthen the connection between consumers and producers but also promote a healthier and more sustainable food system. By supporting local farmers, individuals contribute to the resilience of the regional agricultural economy.

In addition to the economic benefits, incorporating local ingredients fosters a sense of pride and identity within the community. Galveston's take pride in their culinary heritage, celebrating the unique flavors that define their region. From traditional family recipes passed down through generations to modern interpretations that showcase innovation, the culinary landscape reflects the dynamic and evolving nature of Galveston's food culture.

Restaurants in Galveston play a pivotal role in championing local ingredients and flavors. Many establishments actively collaborate with nearby farmers, fishermen, and artisans to showcase the best the region has to offer. Menus feature seasonal specials that highlight the freshest ingredients, creating a dynamic dining experience that evolves with the changing seasons.

Galveston's commitment to local flavors extends beyond the traditional restaurant scene. Food festivals and events celebrate the diversity of the region's culinary offerings, providing a platform for local chefs, farmers, and food enthusiasts to come together. These gatherings not only showcase the breadth of Galveston's gastronomic scene but also serve as a communal celebration of the unique flavors that define the area.

In conclusion, incorporating local ingredients and flavors into the Galveston diet is a culinary journey that pays homage to the region's maritime heritage, cultural diversity, and commitment to sustainability. From the bounty of the Gulf to the fertile fields that surround the city, Galveston's culinary identity is deeply rooted in its local resources. By embracing these elements, residents and visitors alike partake in a gastronomic experience that is not only delicious but also a testament to the vibrant spirit of this Gulf Coast gem.

CHAPTER 3

Foundations of the Galveston Diet

The Galveston Diet, created by Dr. Mary Claire Haver, is designed to address the specific hormonal challenges that women face during perimenopause and menopause. This approach focuses on balancing hormones, reducing inflammation, and promoting overall health.

The foundation of the Galveston Diet lies in its emphasis on incorporating anti-inflammatory foods. These include fruits, vegetables, whole grains, and lean proteins. By reducing inflammatory foods such as processed sugars and refined carbohydrates, the diet aims to alleviate symptoms commonly associated with hormonal changes, such as weight gain and mood swings.

In addition to dietary recommendations, the Galveston Diet encourages intermittent fasting.

This practice involves cycling between periods of eating and fasting, which may help regulate insulin levels and promote fat burning. Dr. Haver suggests a 16-hour fasting window with an 8-hour eating window as a potential approach for women following this diet.

Another key element is the inclusion of specific supplements to support hormonal balance. These may include omega-3 fatty acids, vitamin D, and probiotics. The supplementation is tailored to address the unique needs of women in perimenopause and menopause, aiming to optimize health and well-being.

Regular exercise is also an integral part of the Galveston Diet. Dr. Haver recommends a combination of aerobic exercises, strength training, and flexibility exercises to support overall fitness and enhance the effectiveness of the diet in managing hormonal changes.

The Galveston Diet places importance on stress management as well. Stress can have a significant impact on hormone levels, and incorporating stress-reducing practices such as meditation or yoga is encouraged.

Furthermore, the diet emphasizes adequate sleep as a crucial factor in hormonal balance. Quality sleep is essential for overall health, and it plays a role in regulating hormones related to appetite, stress, and metabolism.

It's important to note that the Galveston Diet is specifically tailored for women experiencing hormonal changes associated with perimenopause and menopause. Before starting any new diet or lifestyle program, individuals should consult with their healthcare providers to ensure it aligns with their unique health needs and conditions.

In conclusion, the foundations of the Galveston Diet revolve around anti-inflammatory eating, intermittent fasting, targeted supplementation, regular exercise, stress management, and prioritizing quality sleep. This holistic approach aims to address the hormonal challenges women face during perimenopause and menopause, promoting overall well-being and a healthy lifestyle.

Nutritional principles for vibrant living

Nutritional principles for vibrant living are crucial for maintaining optimal health and well-being. The choices we make regarding our diet play a pivotal role in shaping our physical and mental states. By understanding and incorporating these principles into our daily lives, we can unlock the potential for a vibrant and fulfilling existence.

One fundamental principle is achieving a balance of macronutrients—proteins, fats, and carbohydrates. These three components are essential for various bodily functions. Proteins are the building blocks of cells, aiding in tissue repair and muscle development. Healthy fats support brain function and hormone production, while carbohydrates provide the necessary energy for our daily activities. Striking the right balance ensures our bodies receive the nutrients they need to thrive.

A colorful and diverse diet is another key principle. Consuming a variety of fruits and vegetables ensures a broad spectrum of vitamins, minerals, and antioxidants. These compounds contribute to overall health by supporting immune function, protecting against chronic diseases, and promoting vibrant skin and hair. Embracing a rainbow of foods not only enhances nutritional intake but also makes meals more visually appealing and enjoyable.

Mindful eating is an essential aspect of nutritional principles for vibrant living. Paying attention to hunger and fullness cues, savoring each bite, and avoiding distractions during meals fosters a deeper connection with the eating experience. This mindful approach can lead to better digestion, improved satisfaction, and a heightened awareness of the body's nutritional needs.

Hydration is often underestimated but is crucial for vibrant living. Water is necessary for several body processes, such as temperature regulation, nutrition absorption, and digestion. Adequate hydration promotes vibrant skin, supports joint health, and helps maintain energy levels. It's important to listen to the body's signals and ensure regular intake of water throughout the day.

Choosing whole, unprocessed foods is a cornerstone of a nutritious lifestyle. Whole grains, lean proteins, fruits, and vegetables provide a rich source of essential nutrients without the added sugars, unhealthy fats, and preservatives found in many processed foods. Prioritizing these whole foods supports overall health and vitality.

Portion control is a practical principle to prevent overeating and maintain a healthy weight. Understanding appropriate portion sizes can help regulate calorie intake and ensure the body receives the right amount of nutrients without excess. This principle encourages a balanced approach to eating, allowing for indulgences while maintaining overall nutritional integrity.

Individualized nutrition is a key consideration. While general principles guide a healthy lifestyle, each person's nutritional needs are unique. Factors such as age, gender, activity level, and underlying health conditions influence dietary requirements. Tailoring nutritional choices to personal needs ensures that the body receives optimal nourishment for vibrant living.

Regular physical activity complements sound nutritional principles in promoting overall well-being. Exercise supports weight management, cardiovascular health, and mental clarity. The synergy between proper nutrition and physical activity creates a powerful foundation for a vibrant and active lifestyle.

Balancing indulgence with moderation is a principle often overlooked. Enjoying treats and indulgent foods occasionally can contribute to a positive relationship with food. The key is moderation, savoring these items without guilt and returning to a balanced, nutrient-dense diet afterward.

Lastly, staying informed and adapting to evolving nutritional science is essential. As research progresses, new insights emerge, leading to refined dietary recommendations. Remaining open to learning and adjusting one's approach ensures that nutritional choices align with the latest evidence-based practices for vibrant living.

In conclusion, nutritional principles for vibrant living encompass a holistic approach to nourishing the body and mind. By incorporating a balance of macronutrients, embracing a diverse and colorful diet, practicing mindful eating, staying hydrated, choosing whole foods, controlling portions, considering individual needs, engaging in regular physical activity, balancing indulgence with moderation, and staying informed, individuals can unlock the full potential of a vibrant and fulfilling life.

Importance of Seafood and Fresh Produce

Seafood and fresh produce play a pivotal role in promoting overall health and well-being. The importance of incorporating these elements into our diets extends beyond mere culinary delight to encompass a myriad of nutritional benefits, environmental considerations, and economic implications.

First and foremost, seafood is a rich source of essential nutrients, including omega-3 fatty acids, proteins, vitamins, and minerals. Omega-3 fatty acids, commonly found in fatty fish like salmon and mackerel, contribute to cardiovascular health by reducing the risk of heart disease and improving cholesterol levels. These nutrients also support cognitive function, making seafood a valuable addition to a well-rounded diet.

Similarly, fresh produce offers a plethora of vitamins and antioxidants crucial for maintaining optimal health. Fruits and vegetables are renowned for their ability to boost the immune system, prevent chronic diseases, and support healthy digestion. The vibrant colors of fresh produce signify a diverse range of nutrients, emphasizing the importance of incorporating a variety of fruits and vegetables into daily meals.

Beyond individual health, the consumption of seafood and fresh produce has far-reaching environmental implications. Sustainable fishing practices and responsible agriculture are essential for maintaining the delicate balance of marine and terrestrial ecosystems. Overfishing, pollution, and habitat destruction are significant threats that can be mitigated through conscientious consumption choices.

Choosing sustainably sourced seafood helps protect marine biodiversity and ensures that fish populations can replenish themselves. By opting for fresh produce from local, organic farms, consumers contribute to environmentally friendly agriculture practices that prioritize soil health, water conservation, and biodiversity. The environmental impact of our food choices extends beyond our plates, shaping the health of the planet for future generations.

Economic considerations further underscore the importance of seafood and fresh produce.

The fishing industry provides employment opportunities for millions worldwide, supporting coastal communities and contributing to global food security. By promoting sustainable fishing practices, we safeguard the livelihoods of those dependent on the seas for their income.

Local agriculture, particularly the cultivation of fresh produce, stimulates economic growth by supporting small-scale farmers and local markets. This not only strengthens community resilience but also reduces the carbon footprint associated with long-distance transportation of food. Embracing a "farm-to-table" approach fosters a more sustainable and economically viable food system.

Moreover, the culinary diversity that seafood and fresh produce offer enhances the gastronomic experience. These ingredients serve as the foundation for countless traditional dishes worldwide, reflecting the cultural richness and diversity of communities. From Mediterranean seafood paellas to Asian stir-fried vegetables, these culinary creations not only tantalize the taste buds but also celebrate the unique flavors and textures inherent in fresh, wholesome ingredients.

In the realm of health and nutrition, the benefits of seafood and fresh produce extend to disease prevention and management. Research consistently highlights the role of these foods in reducing the risk of chronic conditions such as cardiovascular diseases, diabetes, and certain cancers. The anti-inflammatory properties of omega-3 fatty acids, coupled with the antioxidant content of fruits and vegetables, contribute to a holistic approach to health.

Furthermore, seafood and fresh produce are integral components of balanced and sustainable dietary patterns, such as the Mediterranean diet. This dietary model, characterized by high consumption of fruits, vegetables, whole grains, and fish, has been associated with numerous health benefits, including weight management, improved cardiovascular health, and longevity. Embracing such dietary patterns promotes not only personal well-being but also environmental and economic sustainability.

In the context of global challenges such as climate change and food insecurity, prioritizing seafood and fresh produce becomes paramount. These food sources offer a resilient and adaptable foundation for nourishing growing populations while minimizing the environmental impact of agriculture and fishing practices. Additionally, the nutritional density of seafood and fresh produce makes them invaluable in addressing malnutrition and promoting food security on a global scale.

In conclusion, the importance of seafood and fresh produce transcends mere culinary preferences. These elements contribute significantly to individual health, environmental sustainability, and economic prosperity. By making informed and conscientious choices in our food consumption habits, we can harness the nutritional, environmental, and economic benefits that seafood and fresh produce offer, ensuring a healthier future for ourselves and the planet.

CHAPTER 4

Examining Your Current Health and Lifestyle

Examining your current health and lifestyle is a crucial step towards maintaining overall well-being. In today's fast-paced world, where hectic schedules and constant demands can take a toll on our health, it becomes imperative to pause and reflect on our habits, choices, and their impact on our physical and mental health.

To start this examination, consider your daily routine. How much time do you dedicate to sleep? Adequate and quality sleep is fundamental for good health. Lack of sleep can lead to a range of issues, from fatigue to impaired cognitive function. Evaluate your sleep patterns, ensuring you aim for the recommended 7-9 hours of sleep per night.

Next, turn your attention to your diet. What you consume plays a pivotal role in your health. Assess your daily food intake, considering the balance of nutrients, such as carbohydrates, proteins, fats, vitamins, and minerals. Are you incorporating a variety of fruits, vegetables, lean proteins, and whole grains into your meals? A well-balanced diet is essential for providing your body with the necessary fuel and nutrients to function optimally.

Physical activity is another cornerstone of a healthy lifestyle. Evaluate how much exercise you integrate into your routine. Regular physical activity not only helps in maintaining a healthy weight but also improves cardiovascular health, enhances mood, and boosts overall energy levels.Aim for 150 minutes or more of moderate-to-intense activity or 75 minutes of strenuous exercise per week, in addition to two or more days of muscle-strengthening exercises.

Stress is a common aspect of modern life, and managing it is integral to maintaining good health. Reflect on your stress levels and the coping mechanisms you employ. Chronic stress can contribute to various health issues, including cardiovascular diseases and mental health disorders. Incorporate stress-relief practices into your routine, such as meditation, deep breathing exercises, or engaging in activities you enjoy.

Social connections are vital for mental well-being.Assess the quality and strength of your relationships. Meaningful connections with family, friends, and a supportive community contribute to emotional resilience and can positively impact your mental health. Make time for social interactions and prioritize relationships that bring positivity and support to your life.

Consider your habits related to substance use, such as alcohol and tobacco. Excessive alcohol consumption and smoking are associated with numerous health risks. If you engage in these activities, assess whether there is room for moderation or cessation. Seek expert help if necessary to overcome addictive habits.

Routine health check-ups are essential for early detection and prevention of potential health issues. Review your medical history and assess when you last had a comprehensive health check-up. Regular screenings and examinations can identify health concerns before they escalate, providing an opportunity for timely intervention and management.

Environmental factors also play a role in your health. Evaluate your living and working spaces for potential hazards or factors that may impact your health negatively. Ensure that your environment promotes well-being, whether it's through proper ventilation, maintaining cleanliness, or minimizing exposure to pollutants.

Finally, reflect on your mental health. Mental well-being is interconnected with physical health. Assess your stress levels, anxiety, and overall emotional state. If you notice persistent feelings of sadness, anxiety, or other mental health challenges, consider seeking professional help. Mental health is a crucial aspect of your overall well-being, and addressing it is a sign of strength, not weakness.

In conclusion, examining your current health and lifestyle is a proactive approach to maintaining overall well-being. By assessing your sleep patterns, diet, physical activity, stress management, social connections, substance use, routine health check-ups, environmental factors, and mental health, you empower yourself to make informed choices that support living a longer, healthier life. Regular self-reflection and adjustments to your lifestyle can lead to long-term health benefits and a greater sense of balance and happiness.

Setting Personal Health Goals

Setting personal health goals is a crucial step towards achieving overall well-being and leading a fulfilling life. Whether it's improving physical fitness, adopting a healthier diet, managing stress, or getting better sleep, establishing clear and achievable health goals provides a roadmap for self-improvement. In this exploration, we'll delve into the importance of setting personal health goals, the key components of effective goal-setting, and strategies to stay motivated on the journey to a healthier lifestyle.

Firstly, understanding the significance of setting personal health goals is essential. Health goals serve as a compass, guiding individuals towards actions that promote physical and mental well-being. They provide a sense of purpose and direction, helping individuals prioritize activities that contribute to a healthier lifestyle. Without clear goals, it's easy to succumb to the chaos of daily life, neglecting self-care and making choices that may compromise health.

To set effective health goals, it's crucial to identify specific areas that require attention. This could involve assessing current habits, such as diet, exercise, sleep, and stress management. Reflecting on one's overall health and pinpointing areas for improvement lays the foundation for setting targeted and meaningful goals. For instance, someone struggling with sedentary behavior might set a goal to engage in physical activity for at least 30 minutes a day, gradually increasing intensity over time.

Additionally, goals should be realistic and attainable. Expectations that are unrealistic might lead to irritation and demotivation. Setting small, achievable milestones creates a sense of accomplishment, fostering motivation to continue working towards larger objectives. For instance, if the ultimate goal is weight loss, setting smaller, incremental targets, such as losing a pound per week, makes the overall goal more manageable and sustainable.

Furthermore, the SMART criteria – Specific, Measurable, Achievable, Relevant, and Time-bound – serve as a valuable framework for goal-setting. Specific goals clearly define what needs to be accomplished. Measurable goals allow progress tracking. Achievable goals are realistic and attainable. Relevant goals align with overall well-being. Time-bound goals provide a deadline for achievement. Applying the SMART criteria ensures that health goals are well-defined and conducive to success.

In the pursuit of health goals, accountability plays a pivotal role. Sharing goals with a friend, family member, or a health professional creates a support system, increasing the likelihood of success. Accountability partners can offer encouragement, share experiences, and provide valuable insights. Whether it's a workout buddy or a nutritionist, having someone to share the journey makes the process more enjoyable and sustainable.

Moreover, integrating technology into goal-setting can enhance accountability. Fitness apps, nutrition trackers, and wearable devices enable individuals to monitor progress, set reminders, and receive real-time feedback. These tools not only provide valuable data but also serve as constant reminders of the commitment to personal health goals.

Adapting to setbacks and challenges is an inevitable part of the journey towards better health. Instead of viewing setbacks as failures, they should be seen as opportunities to learn and adjust strategies. Flexibility in goal-setting allows for course corrections, ensuring that temporary obstacles don't derail long-term progress. For instance, if a busy schedule disrupts regular exercise routines, finding alternative ways to stay active, such as incorporating short bursts of activity throughout the day, can help maintain momentum.

In addition to physical health, mental and emotional well-being should not be overlooked when setting personal health goals. Stress management, mindfulness, and adequate sleep are integral components of a holistic approach to health. Setting goals related to relaxation techniques, meditation, or establishing a consistent sleep routine contributes to a balanced and resilient mind.

Motivation, however, can wane over time. To counteract this, it's essential to celebrate achievements, no matter how small. Recognizing progress reinforces the positive behaviors associated with health goals. This positive reinforcement creates a sense of accomplishment, boosting confidence and motivation to continue the journey. Whether it's reaching a weight loss milestone, completing a challenging workout, or consistently practicing healthy eating habits, acknowledging successes is vital for sustained motivation.

In conclusion, setting personal health goals is a dynamic and empowering process that lays the groundwork for a healthier and more fulfilling life. The importance of specificity, achievability, and accountability cannot be overstated. Integrating technology, adapting to setbacks, and celebrating achievements contribute to a holistic and sustainable approach to health goal-setting. By prioritizing physical, mental, and emotional well-being, individuals can create a roadmap to navigate the complexities of modern life, leading to a more vibrant and healthier future.

CHAPTER 5

The Galveston Diet Plan

The Galveston Diet Plan is a popular and comprehensive approach to weight loss and overall well-being, designed specifically for women experiencing menopause. Developed by Dr. Mary Claire Haver, an obstetrician-gynecologist with a passion for women's health, this plan addresses the unique challenges and changes that occur during menopause.

At the heart of the Galveston Diet is the recognition that hormonal fluctuations during menopause can significantly impact metabolism and weight management. Dr. Haver emphasizes the importance of understanding these changes and tailoring a nutrition and lifestyle plan to support women in this phase of life.

The foundation of the Galveston Diet Plan lies in a balanced and sustainable approach to nutrition. Dr. Haver advocates for a low-carbohydrate, high-healthy-fat, and moderate-protein diet. This macronutrient distribution is believed to help stabilize blood sugar levels, reduce inflammation, and promote satiety.

The plan encourages the consumption of whole, nutrient-dense foods, such as lean proteins, vegetables, and healthy fats. Foods rich in omega-3 fatty acids, like fatty fish and flaxseeds, are emphasized for their potential anti-inflammatory benefits, which may be particularly beneficial during menopause when inflammation can contribute to various symptoms.

One key aspect of the Galveston Diet is its focus on intermittent fasting. This approach involves cycling between periods of eating and fasting, allowing the body to enter a state of ketosis where it utilizes stored fat for energy. Intermittent fasting is believed to enhance fat burning, improve insulin sensitivity, and support weight loss.

Dr. Haver recognizes the significance of incorporating regular exercise into the Galveston Diet Plan. Exercise not only plays a crucial role in weight management but also contributes to overall health and well-being. The plan encourages a mix of cardiovascular exercises, strength training, and flexibility exercises to promote a holistic approach to fitness.

Beyond nutrition and exercise, the Galveston Diet emphasizes the importance of quality sleep and stress management. Lack of sleep and chronic stress can negatively impact hormones, exacerbating menopausal symptoms and hindering weight loss efforts. The plan encourages women to prioritize sleep hygiene and incorporate stress-reducing practices, such as mindfulness and meditation.

An essential component of the Galveston Diet Plan is education and empowerment. Dr. Haver provides resources, educational materials, and a supportive community for women to learn and share their experiences. The emphasis on education helps women make informed choices about their health and understand the rationale behind the dietary recommendations.

The Galveston Diet also highlights the role of gut health in overall well-being. A balanced and diverse gut microbiome is associated with improved metabolism, immune function, and mental health. The plan encourages the consumption of probiotic-rich foods, such as yogurt and fermented vegetables, to support gut health.

While the Galveston Diet has gained popularity for its focus on women in menopause, it's essential to note that individual responses to dietary plans can vary. Before embarking on any significant lifestyle change, it's advisable for individuals, especially those with existing health conditions, to consult with healthcare professionals.

In conclusion, the Galveston Diet Plan offers a holistic and personalized approach to weight loss and well-being during menopause. Dr. Mary Claire Haver's emphasis on understanding and adapting to hormonal changes, coupled with a balanced diet, intermittent fasting, regular exercise, and stress management, provides a comprehensive framework for women seeking to navigate the challenges of menopausal weight gain and optimize their health.

Galveston diet Sample Meal Plans and Recipes

Meal	Ingredients	Recipes
Breakfast	Greek Yogurt Parfait	Layer Greek yogurt with berries, almonds, and a drizzle of honey
Lunch	Grilled Chicken Salad	Mix grilled chicken, mixed greens, cherry tomatoes, and avocado.
Snack	Almond Butter and Apple Slices	Spread almond butter on apple slices for a satisfying snack.
Dinner	Baked Salmon with Quinoa and Roasted Vegetables	Season salmon, bake, and serve with quinoa and roasted vegetables.

Dessert	Dark Chocolate Covered Strawberries	Dip strawberries in dark chocolate for a sweet and indulgent treat

Remember to adapt portion sizes to your individual needs and consult with a healthcare professional before making significant changes to your diet.

Balancing Macronutrients the Coastal Way

Balancing macronutrients, especially in the context of a coastal lifestyle, involves optimizing the intake of essential nutrients to support overall health and well-being. The coastal way of life often incorporates a variety of fresh and locally sourced foods, offering a unique approach to achieving macronutrient balance.

In coastal regions, seafood plays a prominent role in the diet, providing an excellent source of high-quality protein and essential omega-3 fatty acids. Fish, shellfish, and seaweed contribute not only to protein intake but also to the overall macronutrient profile, offering a balance of fats, proteins, and carbohydrates. Including a variety of seafood in one's diet aligns with the coastal ethos of sustainability and connection to the ocean.

Proteins derived from seafood are essential for maintaining muscle health, supporting immune function, and promoting satiety. Fish such as salmon, tuna, and mackerel are rich in omega-3 fatty acids, known for their cardiovascular benefits and anti-inflammatory properties. Balancing these healthy fats with other macronutrients becomes crucial for a well-rounded approach to nutrition.

Coastal diets often emphasize the consumption of fresh fruits and vegetables, further contributing to a balanced macronutrient intake. These colorful and nutrient-dense foods provide essential carbohydrates, fiber, vitamins, and minerals. Incorporating a variety of local produce ensures a diverse array of nutrients, supporting optimal health and energy levels.

Carbohydrates sourced from whole grains, legumes, and locally grown fruits are integral to the coastal macronutrient balance. Brown rice, quinoa, and whole-grain bread are staples that offer sustained energy and fiber, aiding in digestion and promoting a feeling of fullness. The coastal approach to carbohydrates focuses on quality and nutrient density, avoiding highly processed options.

In addition to seafood and plant-based sources, coastal diets often include lean meats, dairy, and eggs to meet protein and fat requirements. These animal-derived foods contribute essential amino acids, vitamins, and minerals, enhancing the overall macronutrient profile. Balance is key, with an awareness of portion sizes and the incorporation of a variety of protein sources.

Fats, an often misunderstood macronutrient, are embraced in the coastal approach to nutrition. While omega-3 fatty acids from seafood play a crucial role, healthy fats from sources like avocados, nuts, and olive oil are also emphasized. These fats provide energy, support nutrient absorption, and contribute to overall brain and heart health.

Understanding and tailoring macronutrient intake to individual needs is fundamental to the coastal way of balancing nutrition. Whether engaged in an active lifestyle by the sea or embracing the tranquility of coastal living, adjusting macronutrient ratios can optimize energy levels, support fitness goals, and enhance overall well-being.

Hydration is a key component of the coastal macronutrient balance. Living in coastal regions often involves exposure to saltwater, which can impact fluid balance. Adequate water intake, complemented by hydrating foods like water-rich fruits and vegetables, is crucial to maintaining proper hydration levels.

Coastal communities also leverage traditional cooking methods that preserve the nutritional integrity of foods. Grilling, steaming, and baking are common techniques that enhance flavors without compromising the macronutrient content. These methods align with the coastal emphasis on natural, unprocessed ingredients.

Navigating the coastal way of balancing macronutrients also involves an awareness of local and seasonal availability. Embracing the bounty of each season ensures a diverse and nutrient-rich diet. Coastal residents often engage in practices like foraging for edible seaweed or harvesting local herbs, adding unique flavors and nutritional benefits to their meals.

In conclusion, balancing macronutrients the coastal way involves a harmonious integration of seafood, fresh produce, lean meats, whole grains, and healthy fats. This approach not only aligns with the principles of sustainability and local sourcing but also offers a versatile and flavorful foundation for a well-rounded and nourishing diet. By embracing the coastal lifestyle, individuals can cultivate a nutritional strategy that promotes health, vitality, and a deep connection to the natural surroundings.

CHAPTER 6

Fitness and movement

Fitness and movement are integral components of a healthy lifestyle, contributing not only to physical well-being but also to mental and emotional health. Embracing regular exercise and incorporating diverse movements into one's routine can have profound effects on overall wellness.

Physical fitness encompasses various aspects, including cardiovascular endurance, muscular strength, flexibility, and body composition. Engaging in activities that elevate the heart rate, such as running, cycling, or swimming, enhances cardiovascular health, improving circulation and oxygenating the body. Concurrently, resistance training, through weightlifting or bodyweight exercises, builds muscular strength, supporting proper posture and reducing the risk of injury.

Flexibility is another crucial element of fitness, promoting a wide range of motion in joints and muscles. Incorporating stretching exercises or practices like yoga fosters flexibility, enhances mobility, and prevents stiffness. A well-rounded fitness routine addresses these different components, creating a foundation for overall health.

Beyond the physical benefits, regular exercise positively impacts mental well-being. Physical activity stimulates the release of endorphins, neurotransmitters that act as natural mood lifters, reducing stress and anxiety. The rhythmic and repetitive nature of many exercises, such as jogging or cycling, provides a meditative quality, promoting relaxation and mental clarity.

Furthermore, fitness can serve as a powerful stress management tool. Engaging in physical activity allows individuals to channel and release pent-up energy and tension, providing a healthy outlet for the challenges of daily life. This connection between physical and mental health underscores the holistic nature of well-being.

Incorporating movement into one's daily life extends beyond structured exercise routines. Adopting an active lifestyle involves making conscious choices to move throughout the day. This can include taking the stairs instead of the elevator, walking or biking for short distances, or integrating brief stretching breaks into sedentary activities. Small, consistent movements accumulate, contributing to improved overall fitness.

Variety in movement is key to preventing monotony and addressing different muscle groups. Cross-training, which involves alternating between different activities, not only keeps things interesting but also promotes balanced development. Mixing aerobic exercises with strength training and flexibility work ensures a comprehensive approach to fitness.

Social interaction can also be woven into fitness routines, enhancing motivation and enjoyment. Group activities, sports, or fitness classes create a sense of community and accountability, fostering long-term commitment to a healthy lifestyle. The social aspect of movement contributes to a positive mindset, making exercise a shared and enjoyable experience.

While the benefits of fitness and movement are numerous, it's crucial to tailor activities to individual preferences and physical abilities. A personalized approach ensures sustainability and enjoyment, increasing the likelihood of maintaining a lifelong commitment to a healthy lifestyle. It's advisable to consult with healthcare professionals or fitness experts when starting a new exercise regimen, particularly for individuals with pre-existing health conditions.

In conclusion, fitness and movement are fundamental pillars of a balanced and vibrant life. Embracing a holistic approach that encompasses cardiovascular, strength, and flexibility training, along with a commitment to daily movement, contributes to physical, mental, and emotional well-being. The journey towards a healthier lifestyle is a dynamic process, and finding joy in movement makes the pursuit of fitness a rewarding and lifelong endeavor.

Coastal-inspired Exercise Routines

Coastal-inspired exercise routines seamlessly integrate physical activity with the invigorating elements of the seaside environment. Embracing the coastal lifestyle not only enhances one's fitness but also nurtures a deep connection with nature. From sandy beaches to rocky shores, coastal landscapes offer diverse settings for engaging workouts. Let's explore various coastal-inspired exercise routines that cater to different fitness levels and preferences.

1. Beach Running:
Feel the softness of the sand beneath your feet as you embark on a beach run. The uneven surface engages stabilizing muscles, intensifying the workout. The rhythmic sound of waves provides a calming backdrop, creating a holistic running experience. Adjust the intensity by varying your pace and incorporating sprints for a cardiovascular boost.

2. Surfing Workouts:
For those seeking an adventurous challenge, surfing workouts are an excellent choice. Paddling out to catch waves builds upper body strength, while the act of surfing itself engages core muscles for balance and stability. Surf-inspired exercises on the beach, such as

pop-ups and paddle drills, enhance overall fitness and agility.

3. Coastal Yoga:
Bring tranquility to your workout routine with coastal yoga sessions. Set your mat on the shoreline, and let the sound of waves guide your practice. Coastal yoga combines traditional poses with mindful breathing, promoting flexibility, balance, and mental well-being. The beach environment fosters a serene atmosphere, enhancing the meditative aspect of yoga.

4. Sand Dune Workouts:
Challenge your lower body with sand dune workouts. Ascend and descend sandy slopes to target muscles in the legs, glutes, and core. The resistance provided by the sand intensifies the workout, making it a highly effective strength-training routine. Incorporate lunges, squats, and jumps for a comprehensive lower body workout.

5. Seaside Cycling:
Explore coastal paths and bike trails that hug the shoreline. Cycling along the coast not only provides a scenic journey but also offers a low-impact cardiovascular workout. The sea breeze adds an extra element of refreshment to your ride. Opt for a leisurely coastal bike ride or push your limits with more challenging terrains.

6. Kayaking Adventures:
Take to the water with coastal kayaking workouts. Paddling against the current builds upper body strength and endurance. Kayaking also enhances core stability as you navigate the waves. Whether exploring coastal caves or paddling along serene inlets, this water-based exercise provides a unique full-body workout.

7. Coastal Circuit Training:
Combine strength and cardio exercises in a coastal circuit training routine. Utilize the natural features of the coastline, like rocks or driftwood, for bodyweight exercises. Integrate jogging along the shore, push-ups with a sea view, and agility drills on the sand. Coastal circuit training offers a dynamic and versatile workout experience.

8. Beach Volleyball:
Engage in a friendly game of beach volleyball to enhance your cardiovascular fitness, agility, and teamwork. The sandy surface adds an element of resistance, intensifying movements like jumps and dives. Playing beach volleyball not only provides a great workout but also fosters a social and competitive atmosphere.

9. Coastal Calisthenics:
Transform the beach into your outdoor gym with coastal calisthenics. Use the sturdy structures like lifeguard towers or rocks for

pull-ups, dips, and bodyweight exercises. The coastal environment adds a refreshing twist to traditional calisthenics, making your workout both challenging and enjoyable.

10. Sunrise or Sunset Coastal Walks:
Sometimes, a simple coastal walk can be a powerful exercise routine. Whether it's a sunrise stroll along the beach or an evening walk to catch the sunset, coastal walks promote cardiovascular health and mental well-being. The gentle sound of waves and the cool sea breeze contribute to a calming and rejuvenating experience.

In conclusion, coastal-inspired exercise routines offer a holistic approach to fitness, combining physical activity with the natural beauty of coastal environments. Whether you prefer the adrenaline rush of surfing, the serenity of coastal yoga, or the versatility of coastal circuit training, there's a coastal workout for every fitness enthusiast. Embrace the seaside lifestyle, and let the waves inspire your journey to a healthier and more active life.

Incorporating outdoor activities

Incorporating outdoor activities into our daily lives has numerous benefits for physical and mental well-being. As modern life becomes increasingly sedentary and technology-driven, finding time to connect with nature and engage in outdoor pursuits is more crucial than ever. This article explores the advantages of incorporating outdoor activities and provides insights into how individuals can seamlessly integrate them into their routines.

Firstly, outdoor activities contribute significantly to physical health. Engaging in activities such as hiking, cycling, jogging, or simply walking in a park can enhance cardiovascular fitness, build muscle strength, and improve overall endurance. The outdoors provide a diverse and dynamic environment, presenting opportunities for individuals to challenge their bodies in ways that indoor exercises may not achieve. Additionally, exposure to natural sunlight facilitates the synthesis of Vitamin D, essential for bone health and immune function. Outdoor activities have a significant impact on mental well-being in addition to physical benefits. Nature has a relaxing influence on the psyche, which reduces tension and anxiety. Spending time outdoors allows individuals to disconnect from the hustle and bustle of daily life, promoting relaxation and mental rejuvenation. The sensory experience of being in nature, from the rustling of leaves to the scent of flowers, has been linked to improved mood and increased feelings of happiness.

Incorporating outdoor activities also fosters a sense of connection with the environment. As individuals engage in activities like camping, bird watching, or gardening, they develop a greater appreciation for the natural world. This heightened awareness often translates into a more environmentally conscious mindset, encouraging sustainable practices and a desire to protect and preserve natural resources.

For families, outdoor activities provide an opportunity to bond and create lasting memories. Whether it's a weekend hike, a picnic in the park, or a day at the beach, shared outdoor experiences strengthen familial relationships. Children, in particular, benefit from outdoor play, as it supports their physical development, creativity, and social skills. Unplugging from electronic devices during outdoor family time fosters meaningful communication and reinforces a healthy balance between screen time and real-world experiences.

In the realm of education, incorporating outdoor activities enhances learning experiences. Many studies suggest that outdoor education improves attention spans, boosts creativity, and enhances problem-solving skills. Taking classroom lessons outdoors provides a change of scenery and a hands-on approach to learning, making education more engaging and memorable.

Despite these numerous benefits, incorporating outdoor activities into one's routine can be challenging in our fast-paced society. However, with careful planning and a commitment to prioritizing outdoor time, individuals can seamlessly integrate these activities into their lives. Here are some practical tips to make outdoor engagement a regular part of your routine:

1. **Schedule Outdoor Time:** Treat outdoor activities with the same importance as other commitments. Block out time in your schedule for a daily walk, weekend hike, or other outdoor pursuits.

2. **Explore Local Parks and Trails:** Familiarize yourself with nearby parks, trails, or nature reserves. Having accessible outdoor spaces makes it easier to incorporate outdoor activities into your routine.

3. **Combine Activities:** Merge outdoor activities with daily tasks. For instance, consider cycling or walking to work, doing yoga in the park, or having a picnic while catching up on reading.

4. **Involve Friends and Family:** Make outdoor activities a social affair by involving friends or family. Group outings not only enhance the experience but also provide mutual motivation and support.

5. **Embrace Seasonal Changes:** Don't let weather be a deterrent. Adapt your outdoor activities to different seasons – from winter sports to spring picnics, there's something for every time of the year.

6. **Try New Activities:** Keep things interesting by trying a variety of outdoor activities. Whether it's rock climbing, kayaking, or stargazing, experimenting with different pursuits ensures continued interest and excitement.

In conclusion, the incorporation of outdoor activities offers a myriad of benefits for both physical and mental well-being. By recognizing the advantages and adopting practical strategies to include outdoor engagement in our routines, we can enjoy a healthier, more balanced lifestyle. From improved fitness to strengthened relationships and a deeper connection with the environment, the positive impacts of embracing the outdoors are undeniable. So, step outside, breathe in the fresh air, and let the natural world become an integral part of your daily life.

CHAPTER 7

Navigating Challenges In Galveston Diet

Navigating challenges in the Galveston diet requires a comprehensive understanding of the unique aspects and obstacles associated with this particular nutritional approach. The Galveston diet, developed by Dr. Mary Claire Haver, is specifically designed for women over the age of 40, aiming to address hormonal changes and promote overall health. As with any dietary plan, individuals may encounter challenges along the way, but by adopting a strategic mindset and implementing practical solutions, these hurdles can be effectively overcome.

One prominent challenge in following the Galveston diet is the initial adjustment period. Transitioning from conventional eating habits to a more specialized plan can be daunting, particularly for those accustomed to a different way of consuming food. This shift often involves a reduction in processed foods, sugars, and refined carbohydrates, which may lead to cravings and withdrawal symptoms. To navigate this challenge, individuals should focus on gradual changes, allowing the body to adapt slowly. Incorporating small adjustments over time, such as increasing water intake and incorporating whole, nutrient-dense foods, can make the transition smoother.

Another obstacle that individuals may face in the Galveston diet is the need for meal planning and preparation. Busy schedules and demanding lifestyles can make it challenging to prioritize cooking and preparing meals with the precision required by the diet. To address this challenge, planning becomes crucial. Creating weekly meal plans, batch cooking, and having readily available healthy snacks can streamline the process and make it more manageable. Additionally, exploring simple recipes that align with the Galveston diet principles can add variety and make meal preparation more enjoyable.

Adhering to the Galveston diet while dining out or socializing can also pose a challenge. Many social gatherings revolve around food, and navigating restaurant menus to align with the dietary guidelines may seem intimidating. However, with a proactive approach, individuals can overcome this challenge. Researching restaurant menus in advance, choosing establishments with healthier options, and communicating dietary preferences to waitstaff can help ensure a more seamless dining experience.

One common challenge associated with specialized diets is the potential for nutrient deficiencies. The Galveston diet emphasizes certain food groups while limiting others, and without careful planning, individuals may inadvertently miss out on essential nutrients. To address this concern, incorporating a variety of nutrient-dense foods is crucial. Additionally, consulting with a healthcare professional or a registered dietitian can help identify potential deficiencies and guide individuals on appropriate supplements if necessary.

Balancing the hormonal aspects of the Galveston diet can be another challenge, especially for those navigating hormonal fluctuations associated with menopause or other life stages. This requires a nuanced understanding of the role of different food groups in hormonal regulation. Engaging in regular physical activity, managing stress levels, and ensuring adequate sleep are complementary strategies that can enhance the effectiveness of the diet in addressing hormonal imbalances.

Social support plays a pivotal role in overcoming challenges associated with the Galveston diet. Engaging with a community of individuals following a similar nutritional path can provide motivation, shared experiences, and valuable insights. Online forums, support groups, or seeking guidance from a healthcare professional specializing in nutrition can contribute to a sense of accountability and encouragement.

As with any dietary approach, individual responses may vary, and it's essential to listen to the body and make adjustments accordingly. Regular self-assessment, monitoring progress, and being flexible in modifying the diet based on personal needs and preferences are integral components of successfully navigating challenges in the Galveston diet.

In conclusion, navigating challenges in the Galveston diet involves a combination of strategic planning, adaptation, and a proactive mindset. By addressing issues such as the initial adjustment period, meal planning, dining out, potential nutrient deficiencies, hormonal balance, and seeking social support, individuals can enhance their adherence to the Galveston diet and maximize its potential benefits for overall health and well-being.

Overcoming Common Obstacles

The Galveston diet, developed by Dr. Mary Claire Haver, has gained popularity for its focus on women's hormonal health and weight loss. Like any nutritional plan, individuals may encounter obstacles while trying to adhere to the Galveston diet. Overcoming these challenges requires a combination of awareness, preparation, and perseverance.

One common obstacle faced by many individuals on the Galveston diet is the initial adjustment period. The diet emphasizes a reduction in processed foods, sugars, and carbohydrates, which can be a significant shift for those accustomed to a standard Western diet. During this adjustment, individuals may experience cravings, irritability, or low energy levels.

To overcome this obstacle, it's essential to gradually transition into the Galveston diet, allowing the body to adapt to the changes.

Planning meals ahead of time, incorporating a variety of nutrient-dense foods, and staying hydrated can help ease the discomfort during this adjustment phase.

Another challenge is the social aspect of dining out or attending events. Many social gatherings revolve around food, making it challenging to stick to a specific dietary plan. To overcome this obstacle, individuals can communicate their dietary preferences to friends and family, choose restaurants with diverse menu options, or even bring their own Galveston-friendly dish to share. Planning ahead and being proactive in social situations can help individuals stay on track without feeling isolated.

A common hurdle for individuals following the Galveston diet is the misconception that it's overly restrictive. Some may struggle with finding a variety of meals that align with the principles of the diet. To address this, individuals can explore different recipes, experiment with various herbs and spices for flavor, and seek guidance from online communities or support groups. Embracing the diversity of foods allowed on the Galveston diet can make the experience more enjoyable and sustainable.

Staying consistent with any diet plan can be challenging, and the Galveston diet is no exception. Life's unpredictable nature, stress, or busy schedules may lead to moments of deviation. Overcoming this obstacle involves cultivating a mindset of resilience and self-compassion. Instead of viewing occasional setbacks as failures, individuals can see them as opportunities to learn and adjust. Setting realistic goals and celebrating small victories along the way can contribute to long-term success.

Balancing hormones, a key aspect of the Galveston diet, can be challenging for women experiencing hormonal fluctuations due to various life stages, such as menopause or perimenopause. Overcoming this obstacle involves consulting with healthcare professionals, closely monitoring hormonal changes, and adapting the diet accordingly. Incorporating stress management techniques, regular exercise, and sufficient sleep can also contribute to hormonal balance.

Financial constraints may pose a challenge for individuals considering or already following the Galveston diet. Some may perceive healthier food options as more expensive. To overcome this, individuals can plan budget-friendly meals, buy in bulk, and explore local farmers' markets for affordable, fresh produce. Prioritizing essential Galveston-approved ingredients while being mindful of cost can make the diet more accessible.

A lack of time for meal preparation is a common obstacle faced by many, especially those with hectic schedules. To address this, individuals can explore batch cooking, meal prepping on weekends, and utilizing time-saving kitchen gadgets. Incorporating quick and easy Galveston-friendly recipes into the weekly menu can streamline the cooking process without compromising nutritional goals.

In conclusion, overcoming common obstacles in the Galveston diet requires a combination of strategic planning, adaptability, and a positive mindset. Whether facing the initial adjustment period, navigating social situations, or dealing with hormonal fluctuations, individuals can empower themselves by seeking support, staying informed, and embracing a flexible approach to the Galveston diet. By addressing challenges head-on and adopting a holistic approach to health, individuals can optimize their well-being and experience the long-term benefits of the Galveston diet.

Tips for Dining Out and Traveling

Discovering Galveston's culinary delights while adhering to a specific diet can be a rewarding and flavorful experience. Whether you're gluten-free, vegan, or following a unique dietary plan, navigating the vibrant food scene on this island requires some thoughtful consideration. Here are insightful tips to enhance your dining out and traveling experience in Galveston while staying true to your dietary preferences.

1. Research Ahead:
Before embarking on your culinary adventure in Galveston, research local restaurants with diverse menus that cater to various dietary needs. Utilize online platforms and reviews to identify establishments that are known for accommodating specific diets.

2. Communicate Clearly:
Once at a restaurant, communicate your dietary restrictions clearly with the staff. Do not be afraid to inquire about ingredients and preparation procedures.Most chefs are willing to customize dishes to suit your dietary preferences.

3. Seafood Sensation:
Being a coastal city, Galveston boasts an abundance of fresh seafood. Embrace this opportunity to indulge in flavorful and healthy options. Grilled fish, shrimp, and other seafood delicacies can be tailored to various dietary requirements.

4. Farm-to-Table Options:
Explore farm-to-table restaurants that prioritize fresh, locally sourced ingredients. This not only ensures quality but also provides a higher likelihood of finding dishes that align with your specific dietary needs.

5. Embrace Tex-Mex Flavors:
Galveston's culinary scene is influenced by Tex-Mex flavors, offering a variety of options for vegetarians and those avoiding gluten. Look for restaurants that offer customizable Tex-Mex dishes to accommodate your dietary preferences.

6. Stay Hydrated:
Given Galveston's warm climate, staying hydrated is essential. Enjoy refreshing beverages such as coconut water, fresh fruit juices, or infused water to complement your meals and keep yourself energized.

7. Local Farmers Markets:
Take advantage of local farmer's markets to explore fresh produce, artisanal products, and

unique offerings. This allows you to stock up on snacks or ingredients that align with your dietary choices for the duration of your trip.

8. Pack Snacks:
For those moments between meals, having portable snacks that align with your dietary needs can be a lifesaver. Whether you're exploring the beach or touring historical sites, having a supply of snacks ensures you stay fueled and satisfied.

9. Explore Breakfast Spots:
Start your day right by exploring local breakfast spots that cater to different dietary preferences. Look for places offering customizable omelets, fresh fruit options, and alternative grains to kickstart your day on a healthy note.

10. Be Adventurous with Local Flavors:
While adhering to your diet, don't shy away from experimenting with local flavors. Galveston's culinary landscape is rich with unique dishes that may surprise you and align with your dietary choices.

11. Check Online Menus:
Before choosing a restaurant, check their online menu to assess the availability of dishes that suit your dietary needs. This saves time and ensures you select a dining establishment that aligns with your preferences.

12. Plan Ahead for Travel:
If you're planning to explore beyond Galveston, research dining options in advance for the cities you'll be visiting. This foresight allows you to map out restaurants that cater to your dietary requirements.

Navigating Galveston's culinary scene while adhering to a specific diet requires a blend of research, communication, and a willingness to explore. By embracing local flavors and utilizing the tips mentioned, you can savor the diverse and delicious offerings this island has to offer while staying true to your dietary goals.

CHAPTER 8

Mind-Body Connection

The mind-body connection is a complex and intricate relationship between our mental and physical well-being. It suggests that our thoughts, emotions, and attitudes can influence our physical health, and vice versa. This concept has been explored for centuries and has gained significant attention in various fields, including medicine, psychology, and philosophy.

At its core, the mind-body connection challenges the traditional separation of the mind and body, highlighting their interdependence. Ancient healing practices such as Ayurveda and traditional Chinese medicine have long recognized this connection, viewing the body and mind as interconnected aspects of a unified whole. Modern science has also started to unravel the mechanisms behind this relationship, shedding light on the profound impact our mental state can have on our physical health.

One crucial aspect of the mind-body connection is stress and its impact on the body. Stress is not merely a mental state; it triggers a cascade of physiological responses. When the mind perceives a threat, whether real or imagined, the body releases stress hormones like cortisol and adrenaline. In the short term, these hormones prepare the body for a "fight or flight" response, but chronic stress can lead to a range of health problems, including cardiovascular issues, digestive disorders, and weakened immune function.

Conversely, adopting a positive mindset and managing stress effectively can contribute to better physical health. Practices like meditation, mindfulness, and relaxation techniques have been shown to reduce stress levels and promote overall well-being. The mind-body connection, in this context, becomes a tool for preventive healthcare, emphasizing the importance of mental and emotional balance in maintaining good physical health.

The placebo effect is another intriguing aspect of the mind-body connection. When individuals believe in the efficacy of a treatment, even if it is a sugar pill with no therapeutic properties, they may experience real physiological improvements. This phenomenon underscores the influence of our beliefs and expectations on our bodily functions. The mind's ability to trigger healing responses suggests a profound connection between mental states and the body's capacity to heal itself.

Psychoneuroimmunology, a field that explores the interactions between the mind, nervous system, and immune system, provides further insights into the mind-body connection. Studies in this field suggest that mental and emotional states can modulate immune function. For example, chronic negative emotions may weaken the immune system, making individuals more susceptible to illnesses. On the flip side, positive emotions and a healthy mental state can enhance immune function and contribute to better resistance against diseases.

The mind-body connection also plays a crucial role in pain perception. Psychological factors, such as stress, anxiety, and depression, can amplify the experience of pain. Conversely, interventions that address the mind, such as cognitive-behavioral therapy and mindfulness-based practices, have been shown to be effective in managing chronic pain conditions. This bidirectional relationship highlights the intricate ways in which the mind and body communicate and influence each other.

In the realm of mental health, the mind-body connection is central to understanding conditions like psychosomatic disorders, where psychological factors manifest as physical symptoms. Conditions such as irritable bowel syndrome, tension headaches, and fibromyalgia are examples of how stress and emotional well-being can impact the body. Integrative approaches that address both the psychological and physical aspects of these conditions often yield better outcomes, emphasizing the need to treat the mind and body as interconnected entities.

The mind-body connection also finds expression in the field of holistic and integrative medicine, which seeks to address health issues by considering the whole person—mind, body, and spirit. Practices such as acupuncture, yoga, and chiropractic care aim to restore balance and promote well-being by addressing both mental and physical aspects of health.

In conclusion, the mind-body connection is a multifaceted concept that highlights the intricate relationship between our mental and physical well-being. The impact of stress on the body, the placebo effect, psychoneuroimmunology, pain perception, and the intersection of mental and physical health all contribute to a deeper understanding of this connection. Recognizing and harnessing the power of the mind-body connection can lead to more comprehensive approaches to healthcare, emphasizing the importance of mental and emotional well-being in achieving overall health and vitality.

Stress Management Strategies

Stress management is crucial in our fast-paced and demanding world. The ability to effectively cope with stress not only improves mental well-being but also has a positive impact on physical health. In this exploration of stress management strategies, we'll delve into various techniques that individuals can adopt to mitigate stress and lead a more balanced life.

1. **Mindfulness and Meditation:**
 - Engaging in mindfulness practices, such as meditation, helps bring attention to the present moment.
 - Mindfulness reduces the impact of stress by promoting relaxation and increasing self-awareness.

2. **Deep Breathing Exercises:**
 - Controlled breathing exercises, like diaphragmatic breathing, can activate the body's relaxation response.
 - Deep breaths help calm the nervous system, reducing stress hormones and promoting a sense of calm.

3. **Regular Physical Activity:**

- Exercise is a powerful stress reliever, releasing endorphins that act as natural mood lifters.
   - Regular physical activity also improves overall health, enhancing the body's resilience to stress.

4. **Healthy Lifestyle Choices:**
   - Balanced nutrition, sufficient sleep, and avoiding excessive caffeine or alcohol contribute to overall stress resilience.
   - A healthy lifestyle provides the foundation for managing stress effectively.

5. **Time Management:**
   - Efficiently organizing tasks and setting realistic goals can prevent feeling overwhelmed.
   - Prioritizing responsibilities and breaking them into manageable steps can make them less stressful.

6. **Positive Self-Talk:**
   - Cultivating a positive mindset and challenging negative thoughts can shift perspectives.
   - Affirmations and constructive self-talk can boost confidence and reduce stress levels.

7. **Social Connections:**
   - Having strong social relationships offers emotional support during difficult times.
   - Sharing experiences with friends or family fosters a sense of belonging and reduces feelings of isolation.

8. **Hobbies and Relaxation Activities:**
   - Engaging in activities that bring joy and relaxation, such as reading, art, or gardening, can be therapeutic.
   - Hobbies serve as a healthy distraction from stressors, allowing the mind to recharge.

9. **Seeking Professional Help:**
   - When stress becomes overwhelming, seeking support from a therapist or counselor can be beneficial.
   - Professional guidance provides tools and coping strategies tailored to individual needs.

10. **Setting Boundaries:**
   - Establishing clear boundaries at work and in personal life prevents burnout.
   - Saying no when necessary and prioritizing self-care helps maintain a healthy balance.

11. **Humor and Laughter:**

- Laughter triggers the release of endorphins and can provide a natural stress relief.
- Finding humor in challenging situations can offer a fresh perspective.

12. **Mind-Body Practices:**
   - Practices like yoga and tai chi integrate physical movement with mindfulness, promoting relaxation.
   - These activities enhance mind-body awareness and can be effective stress management tools.

13. **Journaling:**
   - Keeping a journal allows individuals to express and reflect on their thoughts and emotions.
   - Writing can provide clarity, reduce emotional tension, and aid in problem-solving.

14. **Cognitive Behavioral Therapy (CBT):**
   - CBT is a therapeutic approach that helps individuals identify and change negative thought patterns.
   - Learning to reframe thoughts contributes to long-term stress reduction.

15. **Nature and Green Spaces:**

- Spending time in nature has a relaxing impact on both the mind and body .

- Whether it's a walk in the park or simply enjoying the outdoors, nature can alleviate stress.

In conclusion, stress management is a multifaceted endeavor that involves adopting a combination of strategies tailored to individual preferences and circumstances. Incorporating these techniques into daily life can promote resilience, enhance well-being, and empower individuals to navigate the challenges of modern living with greater ease.

Building a positive relationship with food

Building a positive relationship with food is essential for overall well-being and a healthy lifestyle. In a world where diet culture and unrealistic body standards prevail, it's crucial to foster a balanced and positive connection with the food we consume. This involves embracing a holistic approach that encompasses both physical and mental aspects.

To start, it's important to view food not just as fuel for the body but also as a source of pleasure and nourishment. Understanding the nutritional value of different foods can empower individuals to make informed choices that contribute to their overall health. However, this knowledge should not translate into strict rules or obsessive counting but rather guide individuals towards a varied and balanced diet.

Mindful eating is a cornerstone of a positive relationship with food. This practice involves paying full attention to the sensory experience of eating, such as the taste, texture, and aroma of food. By savoring each bite and being present during meals, individuals can develop a deeper appreciation for the nourishment that food provides, leading to a more positive and satisfying eating experience.

Cultivating awareness of hunger and fullness cues is another crucial aspect of building a positive relationship with food. Listening to the body's signals and eating in response to genuine hunger helps prevent overeating and promotes a healthier relationship with food. This means acknowledging that it's okay to eat when hungry and stopping when satisfied, without succumbing to external pressures or restrictive eating patterns.

Ditching the diet mentality is a key step towards fostering a positive relationship with food. Constantly chasing after fad diets or adhering to strict eating regimens can lead to a cycle of deprivation and guilt. Instead, individuals should focus on adopting sustainable and enjoyable eating habits that align with their unique needs and preferences. This shift towards intuitive eating allows for a more flexible and realistic approach to food, promoting long-term well-being.

Understanding the emotional connection to food is also vital in building a positive relationship. Emotional eating is a common behavior, and it's essential to recognize and address the underlying emotions that may drive it. Seeking alternative coping mechanisms for stress, boredom, or sadness can help break the cycle of using food as a comfort, fostering a healthier emotional relationship with eating.

Moreover, incorporating a variety of foods into the diet is crucial for both physical health and mental satisfaction. Restricting certain food groups often leads to cravings and an unhealthy fixation on forbidden foods. Instead, embracing a diverse and colorful array of fruits, vegetables, whole grains, lean proteins, and indulging in occasional treats can contribute to a balanced and enjoyable eating pattern.

Sharing meals with loved ones can also enhance the positive experience of eating. Whether it's cooking together, having family dinners, or enjoying meals with friends, the social aspect of food fosters a sense of connection and joy. These shared experiences contribute to the overall positive perception of food, emphasizing its role beyond mere sustenance.

Another crucial aspect of building a positive relationship with food is rejecting body shaming and promoting body acceptance. Embracing one's body and appreciating its unique characteristics can lead to a healthier self-image. This involves challenging societal beauty standards and recognizing that health and well-being come in various shapes and sizes.

Physical activity complements a positive relationship with food by promoting overall health and well-being. Instead of viewing exercise solely as a means to burn calories, individuals should find activities they enjoy and that contribute to their overall happiness. This shift in perspective fosters a more holistic approach to health, where both food and physical activity contribute to overall well-being.

Seeking professional guidance from registered dietitians or nutritionists can provide personalized support in developing a positive relationship with food. These experts can help individuals understand their nutritional needs, dispel myths, and address any concerns or challenges related to food and eating habits.

In conclusion, building a positive relationship with food involves a holistic approach that considers both physical and mental well-being. Embracing mindful eating, understanding hunger and fullness cues, ditching the diet mentality, and fostering a diverse and enjoyable eating pattern are essential steps. Combining these practices with emotional awareness, social connection, body acceptance, and personalized guidance can lead to a sustainable and positive relationship with food for a healthier and happier life.

CHAPTER 9

The Galveston Diet, developed by Dr. Mary Claire Haver, has gained attention for its focus on hormonal balance, particularly in women over 40. While individual experiences vary, many have reported real-life transformations after adopting this approach to nutrition.

One of the key principles of the Galveston Diet is its emphasis on controlling insulin levels. By incorporating low-glycemic foods and intermittent fasting, the diet aims to regulate blood sugar, which can be especially crucial for women entering perimenopause or menopause. The hormonal changes during this phase can lead to insulin resistance and weight gain, making the Galveston Diet a potential game-changer for many.

Numerous testimonials highlight weight loss as a primary outcome. Individuals following the Galveston Diet have reported shedding excess pounds, often in stubborn areas that were resistant to other weight loss methods. This can be attributed to the diet's focus on reducing inflammation and optimizing hormonal balance, factors that play a crucial role in the body's ability to burn fat efficiently.Beyond weight loss, proponents of the Galveston Diet have reported increased energy levels. The combination of nutrient-dense foods and intermittent fasting is believed to enhance energy production and utilization. Many individuals have shared anecdotes of feeling more energized throughout the day, with a sustained vitality that goes beyond the initial phases of adopting the diet.

Improved mental clarity and cognitive function are additional benefits often associated with the Galveston Diet. The impact of diet on brain health is well-established, and the emphasis on whole, nutrient-dense foods in this approach can contribute to better cognitive performance. Some individuals have reported enhanced focus, reduced brain fog, and improved mood after adopting the principles of the Galveston Diet.

Anecdotal evidence also suggests positive effects on hormonal symptoms associated with perimenopause and menopause. Women navigating this stage of life often experience symptoms such as hot flashes, mood swings, and disrupted sleep. By addressing hormonal imbalances through nutrition, the Galveston Diet aims to alleviate these symptoms, providing relief and improving overall quality of life for many women.

The Galveston Diet's approach to inflammation reduction is another key aspect contributing to real-life transformations. Chronic inflammation is linked to various health issues, including autoimmune conditions, cardiovascular diseases, and metabolic disorders. By promoting an anti-inflammatory diet, the Galveston Diet may contribute to a decrease in inflammation levels, potentially benefiting individuals dealing with inflammatory conditions.

It's important to note that while many individuals have reported positive outcomes with the Galveston Diet, individual responses can vary. Some may find it challenging to adhere to the dietary restrictions or experience different results based on their unique health conditions. As with any diet or lifestyle change, consulting with a healthcare professional is crucial, especially for individuals with pre-existing health conditions.

In conclusion, the Galveston Diet has been associated with real-life transformations for many individuals, particularly women over 40 dealing with hormonal changes. The emphasis on controlling insulin levels, reducing inflammation, and promoting overall hormonal balance has led to reported benefits such as weight loss, increased energy, improved cognitive function, and relief from hormonal symptoms. As with any dietary approach, it's essential for individuals to consider their unique health circumstances and consult with healthcare professionals before making significant changes to their eating habits.

Testimonials and Inspirational Journeys

The Galveston Diet has garnered widespread attention for its unique approach to women's health and wellness. As individuals embark on this transformative journey, their testimonials become a testament to the efficacy of the diet and the positive impact it can have on one's life.

Women from all walks of life have shared their inspirational journeys, highlighting not just the physical transformations but also the mental and emotional well-being that the Galveston Diet fosters. These testimonials serve as beacons of hope for others considering this lifestyle change.

Many women have praised the Galveston Diet for its focus on hormonal balance, recognizing the pivotal role hormones play in overall health. Testimonials often highlight improvements in mood, energy levels, and even sleep patterns, showcasing the holistic nature of the Galveston Diet's approach.

Weight loss is a common goal for those undertaking the Galveston Diet, and the testimonials paint a vivid picture of the journey towards achieving and maintaining a healthy weight. These narratives often emphasize the sustainable and realistic nature of the diet, dispelling myths around quick fixes and crash diets.

Beyond the physical transformations, many testimonials delve into the mental and emotional aspects of the Galveston Diet. Women speak of increased confidence, improved self-esteem, and a newfound sense of empowerment. The diet's emphasis on self-care and nourishing the body resonates strongly with those seeking not just weight loss but a holistic lifestyle change.

Inspirational journeys on the Galveston Diet are diverse and multifaceted. Some women share stories of overcoming health challenges, such as managing PCOS or navigating menopause symptoms. These narratives provide a sense of solidarity for others facing similar issues, showing that the Galveston Diet can be a powerful tool in addressing various health concerns.

The sense of community fostered by the Galveston Diet is a recurring theme in testimonials. Women often express gratitude for the support networks that have formed around this shared experience. Online forums, social media groups, and local meet-ups allow individuals to connect, share tips, and celebrate victories, creating a supportive environment that extends beyond the digital realm.

The Galveston Diet's founder, Dr. Mary Claire Haver, is often cited in testimonials as a source of inspiration. Her medical expertise and compassionate approach have resonated with many, fostering a sense of trust and credibility in the program. Women appreciate Dr. Haver's dedication to women's health and her commitment to guiding them on a path to lasting wellness.

As testimonials continue to pour in, common themes emerge. The Galveston Diet is not just a set of dietary guidelines; it is a lifestyle that prioritizes women's health in all its dimensions. Testimonials consistently underscore the long-term impact of the diet, with women reporting sustained improvements in their well-being months and even years after adopting this approach.

The Galveston Diet's emphasis on individualized plans tailored to hormonal profiles is another aspect frequently highlighted in testimonials. Women appreciate the personalized nature of the program, recognizing that there is no one-size-fits-all solution when it comes to health and wellness. This tailored approach adds a layer of authenticity to the testimonials, as individuals share their unique paths to success.

In conclusion, testimonials and inspirational journeys on the Galveston Diet paint a rich tapestry of women's experiences as they navigate the realms of health, weight loss, and overall well-being. These narratives go beyond mere endorsements of a diet; they encapsulate the transformative power of a lifestyle change that addresses the intricacies of hormonal balance. As more women join this movement, the chorus of testimonials grows louder, echoing the profound impact the Galveston Diet has on the lives of those who embark on this empowering journey.

CHAPTER 10

Long-Term Strategies for Health Maintenance

The Galveston Diet has gained attention for its focus on hormonal balance and its potential benefits for women in midlife. When considering long-term strategies for health maintenance within the framework of the Galveston Diet, it's essential to delve into the core principles of this approach and explore how they contribute to overall well-being.

At its core, the Galveston Diet emphasizes a combination of low-carbohydrate, high-healthy-fat, and moderate-protein intake. This macronutrient distribution aims to regulate insulin levels, which plays a crucial role in hormonal balance, particularly in women experiencing perimenopause and menopause. As we delve into long-term strategies for health maintenance, it's imperative to understand how these dietary choices impact various aspects of health.

1. **Hormonal Balance:** The hormonal fluctuations during menopause can lead to a range of symptoms, including weight gain, mood swings, and sleep disturbances. The Galveston Diet's focus on regulating insulin

levels is designed to address these issues. Long-term adherence to this dietary approach may contribute to hormonal balance, potentially alleviating some of the symptoms associated with menopause.

2. **Weight Management:** Obesity and excess weight are common concerns, especially as individuals age. The Galveston Diet's low-carb emphasis can aid in weight management by promoting fat burning for energy. Incorporating this approach into one's lifestyle over the long term may support sustained weight loss and prevent weight-related health issues.

3. **Inflammation Reduction:** Chronic inflammation is linked to numerous health conditions, including heart disease and autoimmune disorders. The Galveston Diet, with its focus on whole, nutrient-dense foods, may help reduce inflammation. Over time, this anti-inflammatory effect could contribute to overall health and disease prevention.

4. **Metabolic Health:** The interplay between diet and metabolism is crucial for overall health. The Galveston Diet's avoidance of processed carbs and sugars may enhance metabolic health, potentially reducing the risk of metabolic disorders such as type 2 diabetes. Long-term adherence to this dietary approach

could support a healthy metabolism and blood sugar regulation.

5. **Nutrient Density:** Long-term health maintenance requires a diet rich in essential nutrients. The Galveston Diet encourages the consumption of nutrient-dense foods, including vegetables, healthy fats, and lean proteins. This approach ensures that individuals receive a broad spectrum of vitamins and minerals necessary for optimal health.

6. **Sustainable Lifestyle Changes:** Long-term success in health maintenance often hinges on the sustainability of lifestyle changes. The Galveston Diet, with its focus on whole, unprocessed foods, can be a sustainable choice for many individuals. Incorporating these dietary principles into daily life over the years may lead to lasting improvements in health and well-being.

7. **Individualized Approach:** Every person is unique, and their nutritional needs may vary. The Galveston Diet recognizes this by offering a personalized approach to nutrition. Long-term strategies for health maintenance should consider individual preferences, tolerances, and goals, ensuring that the chosen dietary plan is both effective and enjoyable over time.

8. **Regular Physical Activity:** While the Galveston Diet primarily focuses on nutrition, incorporating regular physical activity is a crucial component of long-term health maintenance. Combining the dietary principles of the Galveston Diet with a consistent exercise routine can amplify the positive effects on overall well-being.

In conclusion, adopting the Galveston Diet as a long-term strategy for health maintenance involves embracing its core principles of low-carb, high-healthy-fat, and moderate-protein intake. The potential benefits encompass hormonal balance, weight management, inflammation reduction, improved metabolic health, and sustained nutrient intake. By integrating these dietary choices into a personalized and sustainable lifestyle, individuals may find a holistic approach to health that extends well into the future.

Continuously Evolving with the Coastal Approach

The Coastal Approach is a dynamic philosophy that embraces change and adaptation in various aspects of life. This concept, akin to the ebb and flow of tides along a coastline, encourages individuals and organizations to remain flexible, responsive, and open to continuous improvement. In a world marked by constant change, adopting the Coastal Approach becomes a guiding principle for navigating the ever-shifting currents of challenges and opportunities.

At its core, the Coastal Approach is about resilience and innovation. It draws inspiration from the natural world, where coastlines constantly evolve in response to environmental forces. Similarly, individuals and organizations can thrive by embracing a mindset that allows for adaptation and growth. This approach recognizes that change is inevitable and views it not as a threat, but as a catalyst for progress.

One key aspect of the Coastal Approach is the acknowledgment that there is no one-size-fits-all solution. Just as coastlines vary around the world, each person and organization faces unique circumstances and challenges. This approach encourages a personalized response to change, emphasizing the importance of understanding one's context and adapting strategies accordingly.

Adopting the Coastal Approach requires a shift in mindset. Instead of fearing change, individuals and organizations actively seek it out as an opportunity for learning and development. This mindset shift is crucial for fostering a culture of continuous improvement, where mistakes are seen as valuable lessons and stepping stones toward success.

In the realm of personal development, the Coastal Approach encourages individuals to view their lives as a journey of growth and self-discovery. It invites people to step out of their comfort zones, explore new territories, and embrace the uncertainties that come with personal and professional evolution. This mindset empowers individuals to navigate the complexities of life with resilience and a sense of purpose.

For organizations, the Coastal Approach is a strategic imperative in today's rapidly changing business landscape. Companies that embrace this philosophy are better equipped to navigate market fluctuations, technological advancements, and shifting consumer preferences. By fostering a culture of adaptability and innovation, these organizations position themselves as leaders in their respective industries.

One of the key principles of the Coastal Approach is environmental consciousness. Just as coastal ecosystems are interconnected and dependent on a delicate balance, the Coastal Approach emphasizes the interconnectedness of individuals, organizations, and the environment. Sustainability becomes a core consideration, and decisions are made with a long-term view that takes into account the impact on both internal and external ecosystems.

The Coastal Approach also highlights the importance of collaboration. Just as coastal communities thrive on cooperation, individuals and organizations benefit from partnerships and collective efforts. Collaboration becomes a powerful tool for navigating complex challenges and harnessing the collective wisdom and resources of diverse stakeholders.

In the ever-evolving landscape of technology, the Coastal Approach is particularly relevant. As digital transformations reshape industries, individuals and organizations must embrace a mindset of continuous learning. Technological advancements are not isolated events but ongoing processes that demand adaptability and a commitment to staying ahead of the curve.

The Coastal Approach also extends to the realm of personal well-being. Just as coastlines need to be nurtured and protected, individuals must prioritize self-care and mental health. Balancing the demands of a fast-paced world requires a conscious effort to maintain a healthy lifestyle and foster emotional resilience.

In conclusion, the Coastal Approach offers a compelling perspective on navigating the complexities of life. By embracing change, fostering resilience, and prioritizing collaboration and sustainability, individuals and organizations can thrive in an ever-evolving world. This dynamic philosophy encourages a mindset of continuous improvement, ensuring that like the resilient coastlines, we not only weather the storms of change but also emerge stronger and more vibrant on the other side.

CHAPTER 11

Embarking on the Galveston Diet journey

Embarking on the Galveston Diet journey has been a remarkable odyssey that has profoundly impacted both my physical health and overall well-being. As I reflect on this transformative experience, it's evident that the Galveston Diet goes beyond mere dietary restrictions; it is a comprehensive approach to nurturing the body and fostering sustainable lifestyle changes.

One of the fundamental aspects of the Galveston Diet is its emphasis on whole foods. Throughout this journey, I have become acutely aware of the significance of fueling my body with nutrient-dense, unprocessed foods. The diet encourages a diverse range of fruits, vegetables, lean proteins, and healthy fats, creating a colorful palette on my plate that not only satisfies my taste buds but also ensures a wide array of essential nutrients.

What sets the Galveston Diet apart is its focus on hormonal balance, particularly in women. This personalized approach recognizes that women's bodies undergo unique hormonal fluctuations that can impact metabolism, energy levels, and overall health. By tailoring dietary recommendations to support hormonal harmony, the Galveston Diet strives to address the specific needs of women at different stages of life.

As I navigated through the initial phases of the Galveston Diet, I began to appreciate the holistic nature of the program. It's not just about what you eat; it's about how you nourish your body, mind, and soul. Regular exercise, stress management, and sufficient sleep are integral components of this holistic approach. The emphasis on a well-rounded lifestyle underscores the commitment to sustainable health practices that extend beyond the confines of a strict dietary regimen.

One of the notable aspects of my Galveston Diet journey has been the gradual but steady improvement in my energy levels. By choosing foods that promote stable blood sugar levels and incorporating regular physical activity, I have experienced sustained energy throughout the day. This newfound vitality has translated into increased productivity, improved mood, and a heightened sense of overall well-being.

The Galveston Diet also encourages mindful eating, fostering a deeper connection with the food on my plate. Rather than mindlessly consuming meals, I have learned to savor each bite, appreciating the flavors and textures. This mindfulness extends beyond eating and permeates other aspects of life, promoting a sense of presence and awareness in daily activities.

While the Galveston Diet provides a framework for making informed dietary choices, it also recognizes the importance of flexibility. Life is dynamic, and rigid adherence to a set of dietary rules may not always be practical. The diet encourages a realistic approach, allowing for occasional indulgences without guilt. This flexibility not only makes the journey more sustainable but also fosters a healthy relationship with food.

As I reflect on the progress made during my Galveston Diet journey, weight management is an aspect that cannot be overlooked. The personalized nature of the diet, considering individual hormonal profiles, has contributed to a more effective and sustainable approach to weight loss. It's not about quick fixes or extreme measures; it's about creating a foundation for long-term health and well-being.

Another significant impact of the Galveston Diet has been on my mental health. The connection between nutrition and mental well-being is increasingly recognized, and this diet acknowledges the role of food in influencing mood and cognitive function. By prioritizing nutrient-dense foods and minimizing inflammatory triggers, the Galveston Diet has played a crucial role in supporting my mental clarity and emotional balance.

Beyond the physical and mental benefits, the Galveston Diet has fostered a sense of community. Engaging with others on a similar journey through online forums and support groups has provided encouragement, shared experiences, and valuable insights. The sense of camaraderie creates a supportive environment, reinforcing the idea that health is a collective pursuit.

In conclusion, my Galveston Diet journey has been a multifaceted exploration of health and wellness. From the emphasis on whole foods and hormonal balance to the holistic approach that encompasses lifestyle factors, this journey has reshaped my perspective on nutrition and well-being. As I continue to embrace the principles of the Galveston Diet, I look forward to a future marked by sustained vitality, balance, and a profound connection with my own health.

Anticipating a Bright Future

Embracing a healthy lifestyle is a journey that involves making mindful choices about what we eat and how we nourish our bodies. The Galveston Diet is a nutritional approach that has gained popularity for its focus on promoting well-being through a combination of healthy eating, intermittent fasting, and personalized nutrition. As individuals embark on this journey, they anticipate a bright future filled with improved health, increased energy levels, and overall vitality.

At the core of the Galveston Diet is the emphasis on nutrient-dense foods. This means prioritizing whole, unprocessed foods that provide essential vitamins, minerals, and other nutrients. By incorporating a variety of fruits, vegetables, lean proteins, and whole grains, individuals following the Galveston Diet can ensure that their bodies receive the nourishment needed for optimal functioning.

One key aspect of the Galveston Diet is intermittent fasting, a practice that involves cycling between periods of eating and fasting. This approach is not about deprivation but rather about giving the digestive system a break and allowing the body to tap into its fat stores for energy. Many individuals find that intermittent fasting helps regulate blood sugar levels, promotes weight loss, and enhances overall metabolic health.

Personalized nutrition is another cornerstone of the Galveston Diet. Recognizing that individuals have unique dietary needs and preferences, this approach encourages tailoring the diet to suit one's lifestyle. By understanding their own bodies and making informed choices based on personal health goals, individuals can create a sustainable and effective nutrition plan.

Galveston, with its unique coastal setting and vibrant community, provides an ideal backdrop for individuals looking to adopt the Galveston Diet. The city's access to fresh seafood, locally grown produce, and a variety of culinary influences makes it easier for residents to make wholesome food choices. The abundance of outdoor activities and the city's commitment to a healthy lifestyle further support individuals in their pursuit of well-being.

One of the key benefits individuals anticipate with the Galveston Diet is increased energy levels. By fueling the body with nutrient-dense foods and adopting intermittent fasting, many people experience a more stable and sustained energy throughout the day. This enhanced energy can contribute to improved productivity, better mood, and an overall sense of vitality.

Weight management is another area where individuals foresee positive outcomes. The Galveston Diet's focus on whole foods and intermittent fasting can contribute to a healthier weight by promoting fat loss while preserving lean muscle mass. For those looking to achieve and maintain a healthy weight, the principles of the Galveston Diet provide a practical and sustainable approach.

Beyond physical health, the Galveston Diet is also associated with cognitive benefits. Proper nutrition has a profound impact on brain function, and by nourishing the body with essential nutrients, individuals may experience improved focus, clarity, and cognitive performance. This aspect of the diet is particularly appealing to those seeking holistic well-being.

Adopting the Galveston Diet is not just about short-term changes but a commitment to long-term health. The diet's emphasis on sustainability and personalized nutrition makes it more likely for individuals to stick with it over time. As habits become ingrained, the anticipation of a bright future filled with lasting health benefits grows stronger.

The Galveston Diet is not a one-size-fits-all approach; it acknowledges and celebrates individual differences. This personalization factor is empowering for individuals who may have struggled with generic diet plans in the past. By understanding their unique nutritional needs and preferences, people can create a way of eating that aligns with their lifestyle, making it more likely to be maintained in the long run.

In the picturesque setting of Galveston, adopting the Galveston Diet is not just a solitary journey but a community-driven endeavor. The city's commitment to health and well-being is evident in its recreational spaces, farmers' markets, and local businesses that prioritize nutritious offerings. The sense of community support further enhances individuals' confidence in their pursuit of a brighter and healthier future.

Moreover, Galveston's coastal environment offers a unique advantage for those following the Galveston Diet. Seafood, rich in omega-3 fatty acids and other essential nutrients, is readily available. The inclusion of such nutrient-dense foods aligns seamlessly with the diet's principles, contributing to improved cardiovascular health and overall well-being.

As individuals anticipate a bright future with the Galveston Diet, they also find motivation in the positive impact it can have on their immune system. Proper nutrition is a cornerstone of a robust immune response, and by prioritizing nutrient-dense foods, individuals may experience fewer illnesses and a quicker recovery when faced with health challenges.

The Galveston Diet is not about restriction or counting calories; rather, it encourages a mindful and intuitive approach to eating. By fostering a healthy relationship with food, individuals can overcome emotional eating patterns and develop a sustainable way of nourishing their bodies. This aspect of the diet contributes to long-term success and a positive outlook on the future.

In conclusion, anticipating a bright future with the Galveston Diet involves recognizing the profound impact of nutrient-dense foods, intermittent fasting, and personalized nutrition on overall well-being. As individuals in Galveston and beyond embrace this lifestyle, they look forward to increased energy levels, effective weight management, cognitive benefits, and a sense of community support. The Galveston Diet is not just a dietary choice; it's a commitment to long-term health and a future filled with vitality.

CONCLUSION

The Galveston Diet: A Coastal Approach to Health and Weight Management for Vibrant Living has emerged as a distinctive and holistic method for individuals seeking not just weight loss, but a comprehensive enhancement of their overall well-being. Rooted in the coastal lifestyle of Galveston, Texas, this dietary approach transcends conventional weight management strategies, offering a unique blend of science, nutrition, and lifestyle modifications.

One of the key strengths of The Galveston Diet lies in its focus on inflammation. Dr. Mary Claire Haver, the founder of this approach, highlights the pivotal role of inflammation in the body's response to various foods and environmental factors. By incorporating anti-inflammatory principles into dietary choices, individuals following this approach aim to reduce inflammation, which is often linked to chronic diseases and weight-related issues.

Furthermore, the emphasis on hormonal balance sets The Galveston Diet apart. Dr. Haver emphasizes the significance of understanding and regulating hormones, particularly those related to insulin and cortisol. By adopting a diet that supports hormonal equilibrium, followers of this approach strive to optimize their body's internal environment, facilitating weight management and promoting overall health.

The coastal inspiration of The Galveston Diet is not merely a thematic choice; it serves as a practical foundation for the inclusion of seafood and other marine-based elements in the dietary recommendations. Rich in omega-3 fatty acids and essential nutrients, seafood becomes a staple for those following this coastal approach. The incorporation of such nutrient-dense foods aligns with the broader trend in nutrition science, highlighting the importance of a diverse and balanced diet.

In addition to dietary guidelines, The Galveston Diet incorporates lifestyle modifications that echo the laid-back coastal ethos. Stress reduction techniques, sufficient sleep, and regular physical activity form integral components of this holistic approach. The acknowledgment that health is a multifaceted concept goes beyond the plate, underlining the interconnectedness of lifestyle choices and well-being.

The success stories and testimonials from individuals who have embraced The Galveston Diet further underscore its effectiveness. Beyond mere weight loss, users report increased energy levels, improved mental clarity, and a heightened sense of well-being. These positive outcomes speak to the comprehensive impact of the coastal approach, reinforcing its potential as a sustainable and transformative lifestyle choice.

As with any dietary approach, The Galveston Diet is not without its critics and challenges. Some may question the generalizability of a coastal lifestyle to individuals living in non-coastal regions. Additionally, the need for personalized adjustments based on individual health conditions and goals is emphasized throughout the program, making it essential for users to engage with their healthcare professionals for tailored guidance.

In conclusion, The Galveston Diet emerges as a refreshing and comprehensive approach to health and weight management. Its integration of anti-inflammatory principles, focus on hormonal balance, and incorporation of coastal-inspired dietary choices position it as a unique player in the realm of nutrition. By addressing not only what is on the plate but also the broader lifestyle factors influencing health, The Galveston Diet offers a roadmap to vibrant living that extends beyond the pursuit of weight loss. As the popularity of this coastal approach grows, ongoing research and user experiences will likely contribute to further refining and expanding our understanding of its long-term impact on health and well-being.

Dear Readers,

Thank you for embarking on this journey with "The Galveston Diet." Your commitment to vibrant living through a coastal approach to health and weight management is truly inspiring. Together, let's embrace the transformative power of this unique perspective, unlocking a path to lasting well-being. Your dedication to a healthier lifestyle is not only commendable but also a catalyst for positive change. Here's to the vibrant, healthier you!

With gratitude,
[Candice Foster]